My Dad Got Sick

JAY PERRY

Copyright © 2018 Jay Perry

All rights reserved.

ISBN: 9781980819721

Dad, we did it.

CONTENTS

	Acknowledgments	i
1	To The Reader	1
2	December 24, 2012	5
3	March 5, 2013	9
4	Team Natural Healing	13
5	Believe That Anything Is Possible	23
6	Friends And Family: Your Crying Shoulder, Or Muted Strangers?	29
7	Don't Remind Your Loved One That They're Sick	37
8	March 6, 2014	41
9	Sincerely, Your Cancer Buddy	45
10	The Little Things That Make The Biggest Of Impacts	49
11	Things Finally Started To Get Bad	59
12	Money vs. Memories	75
13	He's Gone… But The Journey Continues	85
14	Please, Don't Forget To Take Care Of Yourself	101
15	What To Do Now	105

ACKNOWLEDGMENTS

This book was only made possible because of the continued support and encouragement from my mom, Kris, Sharon, Hayden, Lauren, Gord Miranda, Ron & Barbara Gondek, Chris Mooney, Dr. Meg Popovic, and Catherine Skinner. A huge thank you to my editor Andrea Dyer for the incredible job and sharing her brilliant mind with me for this project. Matti Haapoja for the cover image. All those who proof read for me. Thank you to the McNally House Hospice, Full-Circle Health Care, Juravinski Hospital, all my dad's nurses and doctors, especially Dr. Frosina and Dr. Juergens for their excellent care and helping us through this journey.

And most of all, thank you dad.
Thank you for fighting.
Thank you for being brave.
Thank you for showing us what love really is.

CHAPTER 1

TO THE READER

Most of us, at one time or another, have encountered tragedy.

If you find yourself in possession of this book, I assume this is the case for you and I'd like to say I'm truly sorry. To be honest, I really wish everything you're about to read were tales of fiction and that my experiences were all a dream. But the stories I courageously share, are my own truthful encounters with life as a caregiver.

This book is an outline of my experiences while taking care of my dad, both physically and mentally, during his battle with cancer. It is a tool designed to help those in similar positions navigate coping, self-awareness, empathy, compassion, self-care, support, education, commitment, grief, love and embracing the day-to-day reality of caregiving.

Although very cancer-specific, these words can provide encouragement to all those questioning whether or not to take on the role of caregiver. I did my best to write the book I was looking for when my journey began in early 2013. I don't have any 'top 10' pieces of advice to offer, and any advice I *do* give is solely based off what was found to work successfully for my dad. I'm not a doctor, and I don't have any professional medical training whatsoever. At the time this story began I was just a son doing everything possible for my best friend – I educated myself on the run.

My dad was given a terminal diagnosis of nine months to a year to live. He ended up passing away two and a half years later, and although he fought hard for us, I want my dad's fight to be worth more. I want his struggles to give inspiration, and I want to see a shy, humble man's battle provide support and hope long after he's gone. I share these stories about a man with an incurable disease to demonstrate how myself and my loved ones were able to extend his life beyond what doctors ever expected.

During my dad's final year, I used social media as a positive platform to share the daily struggles and absolute joys I was constantly faced with. The

TO THE READER

outpouring of love and support I received is what made me realize this book needed to be written.

For obvious reasons, I hate the fact that this book has grounds to exist, but I will use it as a vehicle to share a journey that will hopefully help you with yours.

CHAPTER 2

DECEMBER 24, 2012

The scent of homemade pierogies, the endless amount of cabbage rolls, and watching my grandfather bread fresh store bought haddock. This was a traditional Canadian-Ukrainian Christmas Eve — the only kind I've ever known. We would gather around the table at my.......

Hold up…..To be honest, I had pages and pages written where I was painting a pretty picture to describe the day my dad had an unusually aggressive coughing attack that hinted something might be wrong (cancer, we soon discovered). Like some sort of fancy published author, I wanted to put you in that room. But why? You don't care about that, and you don't care about my dad (don't worry - no offense taken. It took a bout of depression to realize it's not the world's job to care about my dad). You have one person that needs all your care and attention right now. You didn't buy this book to get lost in some fantasy world. You bought it because you want to know what the hell myself, my dad, and my loved ones did to prove science wrong, the ups and downs coming your way and what to expect as a caregiver. And believe me, I know how time consuming being a caregiver can be, so I did my best to keep this book short. I will always get straight to the point, as quickly as possible.

So here we go… your journey as a caregiver isn't going to be easy, but that doesn't mean it can't be filled with many moments of happiness.

This book exists because of one unfortunate reason: my dad died. My best friend and role model was a man of few words, but one with a giant heart. On December 24, 2012, my dad had a coughing attack which led to a hospital visit a few days later where an x-ray showed a spot on his lungs. Upon further investigation, it was determined that he had Small-Cell Lung Cancer. I was crushed. Heroes aren't supposed to get hurt. They're supposed to be invincible.

Motivated and eager to fight, my dad was ready to battle this disease head on… only to encounter another setback. More scans showed that this dumb cancer had spread to his brain: there were tumors all over. He was now deemed Stage 4. *OK, cool… let's fight it*, I thought to myself. But after a few Google searches, I quickly discovered the severity behind when a doctor uses "Stage 4" to describe a situation. The research triggered tears in my eyes.

This was the man who gave up so much to provide the amazing life that I have: the person who gave up his free time so I could play hockey, the man that made me French toast every Sunday morning growing up. Right then and there, I made the easy decision to stop working, and at 31 years old, I decided to live at home with my parents so I could take care of – and spend time with – my dad. I was running my own business and it was starting to take off, but I didn't care. I knew I could always make money. It was now time for a new fight. I was going to do everything I could to help my dad beat this cancer. It felt like I had the disease just as much as he did. This was my mission and I wasn't going to lose.

It was now February 2013, and my dad could finally start treatment. Radiation was performed on his brain before he could tackle the lung. We were all still up in the air on how serious this was, but my dad stayed positive. I, however, was secretly brought to tearful emotions night after night.

Let's talk for a second about the feeling I had in my stomach; the one that feels as though it's ripping your insides out. It stops you from eating. It stops you from sleeping. It's called 'the fear of the unknown' and I hated every second of it. I know what you might be going through right now and I wish I could tell you that this feeling goes away. For me, it stuck around for a few months and only started to fade once a plan of attack was in place for my dad's battle. It also faded when I was spending time with him, but every once and awhile, it would make an appearance. Just know that you might also experience something similar and that this is very normal. Do your best not to fight it, and instead accept that it's there. Use it to motivate yourself to spend time with your loved one.

CHAPTER 3

MARCH 5, 2013

I should have known by the cold weather that this day wasn't going to end well. My dad had an appointment to see his doctors for an update about his progress. I put on a fresh, glowing red v-neck tee shirt that still had the price tag on it, gathered our paperwork, and we headed off. My mom accompanied us to this appointment as well and I'm sure we all shared a nervous feeling that would take over our bodies. As we entered the examination room, we were greeted by a team of doctors. Although looking cheerful, they didn't waste any time in breaking the bad news to us. We were told that the cancer was worse than they originally thought – that it was incurable. My stomach sank, but still not completely educated, I held on to some hope. The doctors said radiation and chemotherapy would definitely help extend his life. *EXTEND HIS LIFE????*, I thought. *No no.... you mean get rid of the cancer, right?*. I knew what my dad was going to ask but I was praying he wouldn't. My dad, a know-it-all, asked that fatal question:

"So how long do I have?"

"Nine months to a year," said one of his doctors.

How they can say that so easily is beyond my understanding. I wasn't sure my stomach could drop any further, but it found a way.

The doctors scheduled an appointment for us to meet with another specialist later in the day, so we had to wait a few more hours at the hospital. My mom wanted to be alone. I had no idea what was going through her head, but I can only assume that she was off crying. Her best friend of 40 years was going to be gone in nine months. I took my dad for a coffee. I can remember sitting at a table, him sipping on that hot coffee, and me trying to be as strong as possible. I was saying things like, "Don't worry…it's just a number" and "We'll figure this out" while holding back my arms from hugging and holding onto him because it might be the last time. I can't even imagine what was going on in his head.

Later that night when my dad went to bed, my mom and I had that discussion nobody wants to have.

MARCH 5, 2013

"What are we going to do?," she asked as tears filled her face. I tried to be as strong as possible, but I couldn't really figure out what to say. The silence that filled the room was the loudest sound I had ever heard. We sat there staring at the ground until I told her that I wasn't going to let him die.

Here is what I learned that day: There will be days full of good news, and days full of bad news. I am forever scarred by that cold day, but I've made sure to take the positive from it. In being told I had nine months to a year left with my dad, I promised myself that I would spend as much time as I could with him. If doctors had said that he had about ten years left, would I have made the best of that time? Probably not. My mindset would have be one of, *Oh, he'll still be here tomorrow.* I urge you: Please, do everything you can with your loved one today. You will regret it if you don't.

I remember this day so vividly. I cried for what seemed like twenty four hours straight. I wanted to trade places with my dad. This was the man who did everything for me and now I couldn't do anything for him.

Wrong.
I could.
I DID.

It took every ounce of my effort, but I made sure to be strong in front of my dad. He always told me that anything was possible, so I was going to do everything in my power to prove those doctors wrong. I was ready to embark on a mission that science told me was impossible. Well you know what? Think again, science!

CHAPTER 4

TEAM NATURAL HEALING

In Western Medicine, the Naturopath is often a subject of controversy. It is an area of healing that is in its early and inaugural stages, but an area of healing that I truly believe enabled me to have as much additional time with my dad as I did.

I've never done any medical training. Heck, before my dad got sick, it was rare for me to even do my own medical research. But I'm about to give you what some might deem as 'medical advice'. Again, as a caution, I have never scientifically proven this. I'm no doctor, and I'm only sharing what I witnessed first hand.

I will always remember what one of my dad's first lung doctors said to us: "There's three things that fight cancer. Surgery, Chemotherapy treatments, and the third thing… well, we don't know. Sometimes we can't explain why people are able to beat the odds." It was the first encouraging words we had heard in weeks. That mysterious third thing is what I like to call hope. And sometimes, hope is all you've got.

Right after my dad was diagnosed, we took him to see a naturopath. Before I continue – if you thought *I* was skeptical, you should have seen the restraint my dad was putting forth. He couldn't understand how some 'hippie doctor' was going to fix him with leaves and magical potions; a harsh phrase, I know, and I apologize to those who are naturopaths because both he and I quickly became believers.

We were very fortunate to have a close friend who had been running a naturopathic practice for a few years, and who agreed to take my dad on as a patient. I believe it was this familiarity with the doctor that gave my dad enough comfort to agree to meet with him. Going in, the doctor knew of my dad's skepticism, so he came prepared with countless studies to show the effectiveness of taking specific supplements. My dad was a numbers and proof person, so this was crucial in winning him over to at least give naturopathy a try.

Our naturopath doctor quickly put my dad on a few things: supplements in powder, pill, and liquid form. These things were to help prevent metastasis (the cancer spreading), boost his energy, boost his immune system, and bring back his appetite. There were many more supplements, but going into specifics about what he was taking isn't what I'm trying to explain here. Every case is situation specific and the above might not apply to yours. Additionally, I strongly caution you to make sure the oncologist or other doctors always know about these natural supplements, and that the naturopath knows the details surrounding the type of disease and ongoing treatments your loved one is enduring. Research will need to be done to ensure that they can mix. In my dad's case, there was never an issue.

As his disease progressed, so did the list of supplements, and so did my dad's patience. I can't imagine taking countless pills, multiple times a day, all at scheduled times. I witnessed how easy it was to forget. He went from zero pills to what seemed like a thousand in a matter of weeks. When someone in your family gets diagnosed with a terminal disease, it's pretty much like the entire family becomes part of it. You all hurt. You all feel pain. But, more importantly, you all need to come together and work as a team to fight this terrible illness.

My dad was starting to lose track of what supplements he took and when he took them. Some had to be taken at a certain time and then others had to be 30 minutes after that. Some had to be on an empty stomach and some had to be on a full stomach. To be honest, it was quite confusing and I was starting to see why people might give up. But I knew that this routine is what it would take. That this is what we had to do to give my dad a fighting chance. So I made a list with checkboxes. I put all his supplements and medications on it. I had headings like 'Morning - With Food', '45 Minutes Later', 'Dinner - With Food', 'Before Bed', etc. Each list had the date on the top so he wouldn't get confused. I even put a colored box next to the supplement, and put that same color sticker on the bottle in case he got confused with the names. After every pill, he would check off the corresponding box. We also had a small timer we would set for those '45 Minutes After' pills so he wouldn't forget to take them. I have no idea what it was like going through what he went through, but I could tell it was extremely tiring and frustrating at times. I needed to do everything I possibly could to make his life easier. So I did just that. In an attempt to make him smile every morning, I would put a joke at the top of each list – usually the dumbest joke ever in hopes that he might smile, start his day off with a laugh, and maybe for one split second, forget that he was in the battle for this life.

To summarize this: I strongly believe in exploring other forms of healing while your loved one is fighting. The doctors my dad had were intelligent beyond words, but they were going off of what was known to them. His doctors said that he would live nine months to a year if he did what they said, because that's what studies have shown. But those studies don't take into account bringing on additional treatments. The doctors won't tell you to do or NOT to do them, because in all honesty, they aren't familiar with them. You can't really hold that against them. This type of thinking is very new. Through my research, it became quite clear that the time medical schools allot towards curative type treatments versus preventative care is small. I was recently at a workshop where a local Gastroenterologist gave a talk on the diet-cancer link, and although it was more based on what to do to prevent disease, he went into frustrating detail about the 15 hours of nutrition training he had while in medical school. He even went as far to tell us about a colleague who developed a full nutrition course and was greeted with a big, "No, we don't have time for that", when presenting it to an educational head. Again, not bad mouthing my dad's oncology team at all. They were so incredible to us and this is definitely not a book to debate the health care system.

Exploring naturopathic medicine was massive, in my opinion, when it came to managing my dad's side effects. The only side effects he ever had from the radiation and chemotherapy treatments were fatigue, lack of appetite (which was soon fixed from our naturopath) and constipation, which – when I explain what we did to fix that – might leave you feeling surprised.

My dad could never fully beat his exhaustion. I believe it had a lot to do with his sleeping patterns. He was having trouble sleeping at night and found himself taking multiple naps throughout the day. Combined with his immune system constantly fighting what was in his body, he was usually tired. But I do strongly credit what energy he did have, to a few of the supplements he was on. My dad became quite the advocate for drinking green tea after researching the high cancer fighting antioxidants it contained, but the mistake we made, and realized too late, was that he was drinking green tea that had caffeine in it. This probably didn't help his troubles of sleeping at night. A decaffeinated green tea would have been a much better idea.

My dad's constipation issue was an interesting one. The day before his chemo treatment, the day of, and the day after, he was to take a few pills that were to contest any side effects brought on by the toxic liquid entering his veins. A side effect from one of the pills was said to cause constipation, which it did. After every treatment, again and again, my dad without fail would be constipated for a few days. He expressed his genuine frustration every time it happened, but he didn't really have any other side effects from the chemo. I was expecting him to be bent over, vomiting in the toilet every night – at least that's what TV told me would happen. We tried stool softeners, we tried prune juice, but nothing seemed to cure his constipation. His doctors would try and up his stool softening medication, and still, no fix. One day I asked the doctor, "What if he just doesn't take the pill that's causing his constipation? He's never had any side effects. Shouldn't we at least try that?". She gave the go ahead and he didn't take that pill during his next chemo treatment. Oddly enough, he didn't have any bowel problems and didn't experience any side effects. If we didn't come up with our own plan to take him off that one pill, he would have had issues after every single treatment.

So, the point is, always question things and never stop researching. Use the internet to search message boards for people enduring similar situations. I don't want it to seem like I'm bashing his doctor, because I'm not. She was so amazing to my dad and our family. But you have to realize that doctors are human beings too and they are often going off of what statistical averages and their education has taught them. At the same time, everyone responds differently to medication and I'm not telling you to take someone off a medication if you don't think it's working. But never stop exploring alternative solutions. The doctors are there to answer your questions and work with you. I truly think that in twenty years we'll all be looking back wondering what sort of crazy liquid we were putting in our bodies to help fight off this disease.

I very highly recommend adding a naturopath to your team of doctors. I know it did wonders for my dad, and to this day, I still very much believe that it was one of the main reasons he never really had any nightmarish side effects. It never hurts to have another professional continually assess the situation and provide medical advice from a different point of view. But to forewarn you, it does come with a cost – at least it did for us in Canada. We were so fortunate that through their work, my parents' medical insurance plans covered all of the necessary chemo drugs, medications, and a portion of the naturopath visits. But what it *didn't* cover was the supplements prescribed by the naturopath. In the beginning of my dad's diagnosis, we were spending an average of $150 Canadian a month, and towards the end, it rose to about $200 a month. That came out of our pocket, but to me, it was a worthwhile expense and the best investment we ever made.

I can't imagine what this time might be like without medical insurance. There was a brief period where my dad's plan was questioning how much money was used, and how much was still available. We were getting worried, so we started looking into different local foundations that offer financial support for cancer patients. Thankfully we didn't end up needing it, but if you do, know that these places exist. There are incredible foundations out there that will help you if needed. I found a few places very quickly with a couple of Google searches. There are a lot of people out there who want to help, you just have to reach out to them first.

Start building a team of individuals, all trained in different fields, to help you with this battle.

On the next page, I have included an example of one of the checklist sheets my dad was using during his journey. That was the dose of daily medicines and supplements required to give my dad a fighting chance.

MY DAD GOT SICK

When Chuck Norris laughs, milk comes out of your nose!

NOV 3 2014

MORNING - WITH FOOD
- VITAMIN D
- ACETYL-L-CARTINE
- MULTI-VITAMIN
- FOLIC ACID
- MAGNESIUM
- ASTRAGALUS

TIME _____

45 MINUTES LATER
- M - CITRUS POWDER

TIME _____

AFTERNOON - WITH FOOD
- ACETYL-L-CARTINE
- MULTI-VITAMIN
- MAGNESIUM
- ASTRAGALUS

TIME _____

45 MINUTES LATER
- M - CITRUS POWDER

TIME _____

DINNER - WITH FOOD
- MULTI-VITAMIN
- ASTRAGALUS

TIME _____

45 MINUTES LATER
- M - CITRUS POWDER

TIME _____

BEFORE BED
- ASTRAGALUS

TIME _____

NOV 4 2014

MORNING - WITH FOOD
- VITAMIN D
- ACETYL-L-CARTINE
- MULTI-VITAMIN
- FOLIC ACID
- MAGNESIUM
- ASTRAGALUS

TIME _____

45 MINUTES LATER
- M - CITRUS POWDER

TIME _____

AFTERNOON - WITH FOOD
- ACETYL-L-CARTINE
- MULTI-VITAMIN
- MAGNESIUM
- ASTRAGALUS

TIME _____

45 MINUTES LATER
- M - CITRUS POWDER

TIME _____

DINNER - WITH FOOD
- MULTI-VITAMIN
- ASTRAGALUS

TIME _____

45 MINUTES LATER
- M - CITRUS POWDER

TIME _____

BEFORE BED
- ASTRAGALUS

TIME _____

NOV 5 2014

MORNING - WITH FOOD
- VITAMIN D
- ACETYL-L-CARTINE
- MULTI-VITAMIN
- FOLIC ACID
- MAGNESIUM
- ASTRAGALUS

TIME _____

45 MINUTES LATER
- M - CITRUS POWDER

TIME _____

AFTERNOON - WITH FOOD
- ACETYL-L-CARTINE
- MULTI-VITAMIN
- MAGNESIUM
- ASTRAGALUS

TIME _____

45 MINUTES LATER
- M - CITRUS POWDER

TIME _____

DINNER - WITH FOOD
- MULTI-VITAMIN
- ASTRAGALUS

TIME _____

45 MINUTES LATER
- M - CITRUS POWDER

TIME _____

BEFORE BED
- ASTRAGALUS

TIME _____

Note: The shaded boxes are actually different colors but could only print this in black and white. This is what I used to color coordinate by placing a sticker on the bottles. The empty boxes are where he would put a checkmark when completed.

CHAPTER 5

BELIEVE THAT ANYTHING IS POSSIBLE

"Those who don't believe in magic will never find it." - Roald Dahl

I'm sure the last little while has brought you to the darkest of places. I can still fondly remember the look of sadness that would blanket my dad's face upon hearing his diagnosis. It is one I will never forget. I will also never forget the look on his face when he was told he wouldn't be allowed to drive anymore: this was when he realized he was in for a fight. My dad loved his car. He loved to drive. He loved the independence it provided him. Not only were the doctor's stripping away his life, but they were also stripping away his licence. This was a hard thing for me to witness. Due to the tumors on his brain, his doctors said he was at high risk of having a seizure and that it wasn't safe for him to be behind the wheel.

Over the course of two weeks, my dad conquered ten rounds of radiation on his brain, and kicked some serious butt! So much so, that the specific oncologist he had for his brain ended up closing his case and handing off all the paperwork to his everyday doctor. The tumors had shrunk so much and stopped growing, that they didn't see them as an issue anymore. The radiation was incredibly effective and gave us such hope going forward. As I said earlier, you will soon come to realize that sometimes hope is all you have. It becomes your best friend and the greatest of tools.

Now here is a quick and true story about what my dad's oncologist once said during one of his appointments. We explained to her that he hadn't had any seizures, headaches, or balance issues whatsoever in that year and a half since his licence was taken. We basically asked if he could get his licence back and how to go about doing it. Her response? "I 100% agree with you. I don't see any reason why he shouldn't be driving, but to be honest, I have no idea how he gets it back. This is an absolute first for me. I have never seen this. Usually a patient with his diagnosis never lives to see a potential of getting their driving privileges back." Instead of being upset that she didn't know what to do, I took it as great sign that we were doing amazing things to keep that engine called 'dad' running, and that we were continuously taking him to uncharted places that kept doctors baffled.

I had to do a ton of research about getting my dad his licence back. Call after call after call was made. He then had to see a few neurologists, tackle more appointments, and endure more tests. After a few weeks, we had the appropriate doctors sign the required paperwork to say they believed him to be safe to operate a vehicle – the rest was in the hands of the ministry.

I want to share a social media post I wrote on October 2, 2014, which shows that anything is possible:

When all of this started, my dad's drivers licence was taken from him because of the tumors that were found in his brain. Getting your licence taken away is like having a huge piece of freedom and independence stripped from you. Since then I call him my navigator as he's been a passenger in my vehicle for close to two years now.

But my dad wasn't happy with his licence being taken away and he knew he was the only one that could change that. He would have to work at this harder than anything before. Never miss a pill, keep doing his treadmill, staying positive and keep pushing forward.

Today was such an amazing day. I got to be a passenger in my own vehicle as my dad drove me this time. He had his licence fully reinstated and is back on the road.

I hope what you take from this is that you should never accept 'no' as an answer. If you want something badly enough, put in the hard work it takes to achieve it. Nothing is impossible. They told my dad that he would never get his licence back. I could just see the look of "oh ya? Just watch me" on my dad's face as they told him that. This is the first time the oncologists have witnessed someone in my dad's condition, get his licence back. This isn't meant to be a dig at the doctors, but just a story of achieving what some believe to be impossible.

This is a small victory in our lives, but it's what we have to take to keep moving forward. I hope you can look at this and keep pursuing what it is you're going after and never give up hope. Small victory after small victory will lead to something incredible. I love to prove people wrong and this is where I get it from. And if you're reading this... just remember that you are meant to do amazing things and deserve it.

Super proud of my dad.

This was something that was never supposed to

happen — the doctors said so. But again, I can't get mad at them. They were going by statistics. But I'm 99% sure those stats didn't take into anticipate the love, belief, and absurd level of determination that my dad had.

I hope what this shows you is that anything is possible. It takes a strong person to have the guts to go for it but it takes a stronger person to be by their side, motivating and believing in them every single day. That person is you. Never stop believing in the power of someone who's filled with hope and love: it's then you can bare witness to the most beautiful of miracles.

The winning smile on my dad's face says it all. He was back behind the wheel. He had won this round of the fight.

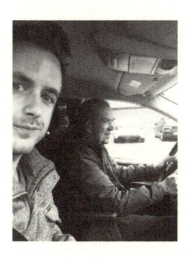

CHAPTER 6

FRIENDS AND FAMILY: YOUR CRYING SHOULDER, OR MUTED STRANGERS?

Can you get through this on your own? Most likely not. I know I couldn't. It was a full year before I made it public that my dad was sick and I still don't know why I waited that long. I was probably scared, and you might say that all the social media posts that came afterwards were a cry for help, or possibly my way of dealing with it. Either way, without friends and family by my side, I wouldn't have been able to cope with everything. But here's the catch: the support I received wasn't from the friends and family I expected.

Now, perhaps putting expectations on others was somewhat selfish of me, but I truly believed that those closest to me would be by my side when I needed it most. I went public with my dad's diagnosis in March of 2014. It's now April of 2017, and I have yet to get a message asking how I'm doing, how my family is doing, or how my dad was doing when he was alive from some people I once called best friends.

The entire experience has definitely changed how I define the word 'family'. I once thought of it as those who share the same blood, and now I consider it to be those who will drop everything to make sure you're OK. It's those who bring you food when you're too exhausted to cook. It's those who come to your aid even when you don't ask. And it's those who label their shoulder as yours to cry on, or who offer their ears to listen. I experienced a close family member almost completely ignore the situation. This was a person my dad thought the world of, and who – in my opinion – didn't use what resources they had to ensure my dad was comfortable and that they would get to spend what time they had left doing things together while he was healthy. It was unfortunate to see, and I knew my dad was probably pretty hurt by it.

I had been spending a lot of time alone. Eventually I knew I needed to get out and see some friends, and that deep down I was just looking for someone to talk to. I had contacted a friend who was performing at a local venue one evening, and was looking forward to talking one on one when the show was over. It was the end of the night, and we were standing outside and the sad look on my face made it evident that something was wrong. That friend questioned if I was ok, either because of my silence all night, or the lone tear coming from my eye. Regardless, that friend could tell something was up. In all fairness that friend didn't know about my dad, but as we were about to leave, he received a phone call from a random girl he met that evening and proceeded to quickly end our discussion to go connect with her as I put myself in a cab and made the solo trip home. It was a really eye opening experience and truly showed me how little value some people place on true friendship.

So what point am I'm trying to make here? There's a good possibility that you might experience this exact thing. The friends you thought were close might not acknowledge your situation. Your family might not either. As upsetting as it was, I don't hold a grudge towards those people anymore. I really believe that everyone has a different way of dealing with things, and sometimes, their way is to ignore it; not to talk about it out of fear it might upset me if they brought it up. They've never been in my shoes and had no idea what I was going through. Or – the harsh truth – maybe they didn't care. I urge you to do your best not to hold any ill will towards people if you experience something similar. It's not worth your time. I know that the close family member I mentioned at the beginning of this chapter undergoes daily regret that they didn't do the things they could to make my dad's situation and his last two and a half years better. It's regret that *they* will have to live with everyday, not me. So there's no point in being upset. What they are going through is much, much worse.

There is a ray of sunshine that comes out of all of this. Challenging times are an incredible way to figure out exactly who your true friends and family are, and more importantly, to meet the new friends that will walk directly into your life when you need it most. I truly believe that you're a product of your own environment and that it's beneficial to be around those who make you happy. Make sure you do that. It's extremely valuable in self-healing. You start to notice the people who will willingly give up their time for you while realizing how quickly money loses value in a situation like this. It's your true friends and family's seconds, minutes, hours, and days that become more important. It's always the most unexpected of individuals who will be there for you. And please, do your best to bottle up your pride and take the help. You will need it.

Take every lesson you can from your current experience, and when it's time, be there for those who need it. To be honest, this is where part of the inspiration came from for writing this book. While I was publicly sharing my dad's story online, from time to time I had friends message me telling me that they had a parent who was just diagnosed with an illness. They didn't say much more than that, but I could tell they were reaching out for help. I wrote them back and asked if they would like to meet up for a coffee to talk, and we did. This happened about four or five times before the idea came to me. Whoever I was meeting would ask what was done to keep my dad alive; what to expect, how they could help their parent. They'd ask what my dad went through, and how I dealt with it. Question after question, I sat there and listened to all of them. I shared my story and offered up my advice. I had lived it and had my experiences to share. It made them feel better and they started on their own journey as a caregiver. I checked in with them every week or so (and still do). After these conversations, I found myself wanting to reach out and help as many people as I could, so I set course to put my personal experiences into words.

I implore you to do the same. Share your story with those who need it. Be there for your friends when they need you and even when they don't. Always check in, and remember – it's OK to ask.

Here is a Facebook post I wrote on February 2, 2016 about this very thing:

With it being World Cancer Day today, I thought I would offer some advice that I think might be valuable to a lot of people.

In short: It's OK to ask.

When I went on that two and a half year journey along side my dad, I had some very supportive friends in my life, but some of them stayed quiet. They never made mention of my fathers illness or ever asked how I was doing. There was no time to get upset at that, and as they say, 'its during the worst times of your life that you get to see the true color of the people who say they care for you'. Although there is definitely some truth to that, I really believe it comes down to them being scared.

I'm sure they question if they even should bring up my dad's illness around me. Maybe they think I'll break down if I start talking about it. So they stay silent. Thinking that silence is the best medicine.

I'm writing this in hopes that it reaches those people who might need it and gives them the reassuring confidence to reach out to their friend going through the same thing I did. Whether it's cancer or any other illness, I'm here to say: it's OK to ask. Not only is it OK to ask, but I recommend it. I can remember the times that friends did ask about my dad. It felt great that they were thinking about us. We were on their minds. There's so much alone time when you become a caregiver, that it's nice to know people are thinking of you. It's a part of life, and it sure is better than sitting in silence.

I currently have a few friends who have parents battling cancer, and every so often, I make sure to check in on them. I know what it feels like to be on that end and how it feels to have people thinking about you.

So I hope this might motivate you to reach out to your friend. Ask how their loved one is doing first, and then ask how they are doing. Send flowers just because. Send a gift card for a restaurant. Our go to response is always: "if you need anything, just ask", but don't wait for that request because it won't come. Take it upon yourself to make your friend's day better, because trust me, every little bit helps.

Miss you Dad.

CHAPTER 7

DON'T REMIND YOUR LOVED ONE THAT THEY'RE SICK

When my dad was given nine months to live, I immediately started thinking about what significant life events he wouldn't be present for in the future. It sucked to even have to think about. My dad – my hero – wasn't going to be there. I felt sadness for myself and I felt even more for him. I knew he was just as upset. After all, I was a single man, and if ever I was to find somebody to share my life with after he was gone, I knew I'd need to come up with a crazy idea to have him present at my wedding with the woman he'd never meet.

I toyed with the idea of sitting him down and filming him. I imagined that in the middle of my speech, on the day of my wedding, I would hit play and the video of him would appear. I wanted him to say something like, "Hello everyone. I'm sorry I couldn't be there today. But I just wanted to say congrats to Jay and his lovely bride. I wish I could have met you in person, but for Jay to want to get married, I know it would have taken someone very special. Even though I'm not there in person, believe me, I'm looking down from above and I'm smiling watching everyone enjoy this incredible day. I wish you all the best." Amidst the tears of sadness that would fill the room, I wanted my future wife to have some sort of approval or recognition and acceptance from the man who meant so much to me.

But I didn't film my dad.

I'm a photographer by trade, so in addition to filming my dad, I also wanted to take a photo of him everyday. Sometimes twice a day. I wanted to capture every last moment I could with him.

But I didn't.
I didn't do any of that.
...On purpose.

And here's why: we've all seen those emotional videos on YouTube that showcase a person's life coming to an end. We've all scrolled through those images on Facebook documenting a terminally ill person's final year. We shed a tear and grieve for these strangers but oddly sympathize with their need to have those last moments captured. My advice to anyone considering this is DON'T. This idea is inspired by the doctor who told us that he didn't understand why some people beat cancer or last longer than science would suggest. I believe that the mind has so many healing properties and that you need to get (and keep) your loved one in the best mindset possible. A mind swimming with the idea that it's sick will constantly find itself on the verge of drowning.

I'm not saying you should ignore the fact that your loved one is sick, but don't remind them that they are. As much as I would have loved to film that video for my wedding, I knew it would have brought on sadness in my dad's mind. We treated my dad as a normal human being. Not as someone fighting an illness. Of course, we made sure he was taking his medicines and supplements, and I took him to his appointments. There was no hiding what he was going through, but it wasn't something that always had to be talked about. I remember in the early days, every morning I would ask him, "How are you feeling today? Did you sleep last night?". Nobody wants to hear that everyday. I truly believe that my dad lasted longer than expected because he was only sick on paper – not in the mind. A positive attitude will go a long way when dealing with disease. It's OK to cry. Heck, I cried.. a lot. But I never let him see me cry.

So I don't have the wedding video or any visible documentation.

But I DO have an extra year and a half of memories with my dad that nobody can ever take away from me.

CHAPTER 8

MARCH 6, 2014

The morning started with a hug. It was the first thing I did when I woke up. "Thank you. Thank you for not giving up," I emotionally said to my dad as my arms gripped him tight. Unaware of what I was talking about, I explained the significance of the day. It was the day the doctors had told us wouldn't exist. My dad was not supposed to be alive on this day. He was given nine months to a year on March 5, 2013. This morning brought him to a year and one day. It was a day I had been looking forward to for the last couple of months. It was a sign that my dad didn't give up and that we were to continue doing whatever it was we were doing. My dad had beat the odds and I couldn't have been more proud of him. As silly as it might sound, it was a time for celebration, and we decided to throw my dad a party.

Ironically, my dad had a chemo treatment that day, but a week before, we organized and invited the friends and family who had made this day possible. We wanted those who had been there for my dad and my family to help us celebrate and applaud the incredible hard work he had accomplished over the last year. Oh – and we wanted to make it a surprise for him.

After every treatment, my mom made sure to have ready whatever it was he wanted for dinner. It was her way of making sure he felt comfortable after a long day at the hospital. Although he was expecting his request of pizza and wings when he returned home, what he didn't expect was the house full of family and friends patiently awaiting his arrival. My dad was a quiet man and didn't love getting attention, so we couldn't anticipate his response. But once he got home and realized what was going on, he had a smile from ear to ear and I could tell he was filled with joy. The evening was all for him. We even had a congratulatory cake made. Congratulations, Darryl. Keep it up. We love you written in vanilla icing on top. Some even brought him stacks of his favorite lotto scratch tickets. There were only a few that couldn't make it but they made sure to call him and say congrats. It was a wonderful night.

This was also the day I first went public about my dad's disease with a post on my blog titled: 'The Blog

MARCH 6, 2014

Post Science Said Wouldn't Exist'.

So why throw a party for a man with a terminal disease, despite my former advice to never remind him about it? Well, I really believe that you have to celebrate the small steps of healing. We wanted to show my dad how much we appreciated what he was doing for us. The endless medication and supplement cycles, the treatments, still exercising, and overnight trips to the hospital. There were probably numerous times where he wanted to give up and I don't blame him. This is why it's important to always show your gratitude for their journey. To let them know, that no matter how hard it is, no matter how much effort it takes, that they are never a hindrance to your life; that dedicating your time and energy towards their healing isn't something you're doing because you feel like you have to – it's because you want to.

I encourage you to always glorify the small accomplishments. Whether it's getting through chemo, finishing radiation, overcoming surgery, or whatever it may be, these steps are all progress towards healing and increasing your loved one's time with you. A body that's filled with love can do amazing things.

CHAPTER 9

SINCERELY, YOUR CANCER BUDDY

You know that moment, where out of nowhere, somebody so important walks directly into your life and makes everything so much better? Thank you, Maggie, thank you.

What my dad was going through day in and day out, I will never fully understand. I'm sure the constant thought of 'Will I wake up tomorrow, or will this be the last time I lay my head down to sleep?' was constantly present in his mind. He never really talked to me about how he was feeling on the inside. He was my dad, and he knew I looked up to him as my hero. Although I would have listened if he'd wanted, I'm sure he didn't want to show any weakness. But how could I offer any sort of comfort or advice if I truly didn't feel what he felt?

Enter Maggie Jenkins: a retired first grade teacher in Bedford, New Hampshire. She was dynamic, loved her students, and was admired by all who met her. She was our family's savior and the one woman who got my dad to open up. Through our family in New Hampshire my dad was introduced to Maggie via email. Maggie was also fighting cancer. They thought it would be good for them to connect, but 'good' is hardly the correct choice of words. It was incredibly GREAT and had such a profound and positive effect on both of their mental and physical healing states. My family is forever grateful for what Maggie did for us and my dad.

It was the perfect scenario for him. He could shield himself behind his computer and open up with somebody who was experiencing the very same pains, and very same emotions. Maggie and my dad would write back and forth all the time, talking about how they were feeling that day, what they were scared of, the discomfort they were having. The list would go on and on. My dad was very skeptical of the idea at first, but very soon he started to really look forward to his emails with Maggie. I noticed he was less stressed, and less worried about his situation. They would sign off each email with "Sincerely, your cancer buddy" and wait for a reply.

I have no scientific proof behind their relationship, but here's what I believe. There's nothing more damaging to your mind and body than consistent stress. One of the best ways to relieve that stress is to talk openly about your current problems. The hospital offered numerous group sessions where patients could talk about living with cancer with highly trained professionals. It was a way for others to see that they weren't alone in this fight. But my dad was a quiet man; wasn't great in public speaking situations, and his social skills with strangers were definitely not first class. So he would never entertain the idea of sitting in a public forum discussion.

Here's my advice: Do your best to convince your loved one to attend one of these sessions. I believe they can be extremely helpful. But if they're on the shy side, like my dad, figure out a way for them to do this via email. My dad found a way to open up emotionally without us knowing. Call it a pride thing for him – call it whatever you want – he was never one to show any weakness, and I'm sure your loved one might be the same. I truly believe these emails were so beneficial in my dad proving science wrong. I think it helped him lose the 'why me?' mentality when he found out how many people are currently in a similar situation, and currently winning their battle.

I will never know what was said in those email

exchanges and I don't need to, but I did go down and visit Maggie a few months after my dad passed to say thank you. Maggie, who was also given nine months to live, was in year three of that diagnosis. A happy, positive, and cheerful woman, also kicked cancers ass. I shared stories about my dad, and she shared how much she loved their emails.

On December 31, 2015, Maggie was taken from us. But not before impacting everyone she knew. We miss you Maggie. Thank you from the bottom of my heart.

CHAPTER 10

THE LITTLE THINGS THAT MAKE THE BIGGEST OF IMPACTS

I have always been a big believer that the only way to achieve the best results, is by having the discipline to perform the smallest of tasks everyday. One's success lies in the consistency of his actions and the belief that what they are continually doing, will not only work, but lead to a positive outcome.

It was a belief I assumed I had picked up from seminars or self help videos until I saw it first hand. It was a drive and determination buried deep into my father's mind that only began to appear when he needed it most. I watched a man take the necessary steps and do those 'other things' that would help extend his life. I want to share those things with you.

Some of these ideas might be common sense, and some might be new to you, but either way: you can only suggest these things to your loved one. It's up to them to decide if they have the will and desire to do it. For example: We currently have a family friend who is fighting for her life. She is undergoing chemotherapy and really struggling. She can't eat, she can't sleep, and she refuses to seek any other help other than what her oncologist recommends. We've tried and tried to get her to see a naturopath. We've cited examples from my dad's journey. But she won't listen. Although the extra steps my dad was taking were effective because we started right away, in my opinion, it's never too late to start.

I believe that a healthy mind can be one of the most effective forms of healing. A healthy mind leads to a healthier immune system, which leads to an increase of much needed healing properties in your body. One of the ways my dad exponentially strengthened his mind and body, was through daily exercise. He wasn't going to the gym everyday or putting his body through hell. All he did was 30 to 45 minutes on the treadmill every morning. He didn't even run. A brisk walk at a pace higher than your average stroll was all he needed to do to break a sweat. We put a treadmill in his bedroom and a TV on the dresser, so every morning for two years, this was how his day started. I don't need to tell you the importance of exercise. We all know this.

THE LITTLE THINGS THAT MAKE THE BIGGEST OF IMPACTS

Heck, everyone should be executing some sort of physical activity everyday. But, what I witnessed every morning was nothing short of awe inspiring. Here was a man with stage four lung cancer, on a treadmill, making *me* look lazy. It became his morning ritual and the importance of doing this came to us from his 'hippie doctor'. It wasn't something his cancer doctors recommended or ever brought up. Please, if your loved one is able, do your best to convince them to partake in some exercise. Maybe even ask them to go for walks around the neighborhood with you. If it takes you having to do it with them, it'll be well worth it.

You can't control whether a person wants to get up and physically move their body, but what you have a little bit more control over is what they put into their body, whether it's medication, supplements, liquids, and/or food. Your loved one's diet is going to become one of the most important allies during their battle. To this day, I get so upset that some doctors don't put more of an emphasis on it. Food is our energy. It's our nutrients. It's what aids in healing. It can also be part of what causes disease. What we needed to do, then, became simple: do our best to eliminate the bad foods, and replace them with good food. Upon my dad's diagnosis, we quickly cut out his alcohol intake, we did our best to eliminate any foods with processed sugars, and we started adding vegetables to all our meals. I've done the research that says to go on a strict raw-vegan diet, and I've also read to stay away from an acidic diet (low pH) and strive for more of a diet high in alkaline foods (high pH). I'm not here to debate the two, I'm here to give examples of what we did. But I do encourage you to do your own research as well. My dad always took his coffee with two sugars. When he got sick we would make it for him, and instead of two sugars, we gave him one. Then we slowly got his coffee down to half a sugar. We would add less and less salt to his food. When shopping, my Mom and I turned into quite the food label readers because if we controlled what food came into the house, my dad would have no option to eat unhealthily. But we didn't go to extremes right away. We eased our way into it as comfortably as possible for him. I felt like taking it slow was the only sustainable way to keep improving his diet and to prevent him from feeling like a test subject for some science experiment.

But oh did my dad *ever* love a rum and Coke. He looked forward to the weekends where he could toss a couple back while watching a new movie. It was one of the hardest things he had to give up, but deep down he knew it was for the benefit of both his health and our family. It's crazy how sometimes it's the hardest of things that result in the easiest of decisions. My dad didn't give up alcohol totally. He found some research that suggested a glass of red wine at dinner every once and awhile was good for you. We checked with his doctors and they were OK with it. I just found it funny that he had been doing his own research, investigating how he could introduce the slightest of cravings back into his life. Eventually it came to a point where any sort of alcohol would have a reaction with the current medication his was taking. He had to stop consuming it completely. Now we all know the negative effects of alcohol on the body, but stripping my dad of a single glass of liquid that could put his mind at ease – and that could make him forget about his situation for a moment – wasn't something I wanted to do. I didn't think it was necessarily the alcohol giving him these positive feelings, but more so the *ritual* of being a normal human enjoying a glass of wine. It was something he had done for the past 45 years. It was the habit that his mind craved. So, here's what I did: I purchased a box of red wine – the one with a spouted bag inside to pour your wine from. I carefully opened the box, cut open the bag, and proceeded to replace the wine inside with a bottle of non-alcoholic wine. I then taped the bag closed and glued the box shut so my dad could once again enjoy a glass of wine at dinner, and pretty much whenever he wanted. He had no idea I was doing this (or at least I don't think he did). He never said anything about the taste, but it made him feel normal, and that was all that mattered.

Dad, if you can read this from up there, I'm sorry

we did that. As much as I think you might have got mad, I do believe you're looking down laughing and smiling because of how much we tried everything for you.

I missed having a beer in the backyard with him. Later in his battle, I eventually did the same with non-alcoholic beer. The habit of holding a brown bottle with liquid inside, was all we both needed.

Here is a post and photo from March 19, 2015:

> *It doesn't matter how sick one might be, you'll never turn your back on the bottle.*
>
> *Killing beers with my Dad right now. Been a long long time since I've been able to do this with him. Best night!*

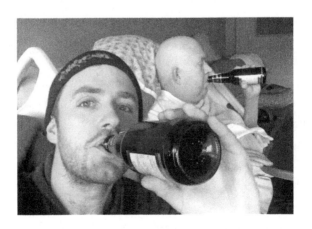

To say what we did next was a marvel of science, would be far from the truth. It's no secret how important drinking water is for your everyday health, but when undergoing treatments, the level of importance becomes raised. Before every treatment my dad had to give a blood sample where he was pricked with a needle, and then again, another needle prick for the chemo injection. That's not counting the other tests, IV's, and you name it. I watched my dad get pricked with a needle over and over. And the more you do, the better chance of your veins becoming harder to find by the technician. To combat this, my dad would drink plenty of water the day before any needle pricks. Staying well hydrated was key for this. Blood is made up of a massive percentage of water. The more water that is in your system, the easier it will be to find your veins and to have a smoother blood draw. There's nothing worse than having to be pricked four or five times by a nurse to find the vein. Make sure you get your loved one to drink plenty of water all the time, but especially the day before a treatment.

I'll keep this next paragraph quick and to the point. My dad's immune system was constantly in a state of battle so we had to do everything in our power to help him keep it up and to avoid possible infection. He couldn't afford to catch a cold, or to get the flu, etc. We always had visitors and different family coming over to the house. Eventually, we realized that they were possibly bringing in harmful bugs that could be passed on to my dad. To try and contest this, we put a bottle of hand sanitizer with a push down pump dispenser (important) at every entrance into the house. As soon as guests entered the house, we made sure to have them cleanse their hands with the hand sanitizer. We didn't think they were always dirty, but weren't taking any chances. I say that the pump dispenser bottle is important because you want to make it very easy for everyone. People are lazy, and you don't want to risk the chance that they bypass sanitizing their hands because they don't want to open a lid, turn the bottle upside down, and squeeze. Sundays soon became 'Sanitize Sundays' in our household. Now, we weren't germaphobes by any means, but we were always cautious of germs and bacteria we might be bringing into our home. Every Sunday, we would make sure all the door handles, light switches, phones, cupboard doors, appliances, remotes, and anything else my dad regularly came in contact with were clean and sterile. This might sound over the top, but if you saw the negative effects a simple cold can have on an individual with a weakened immune system, you would do the same.

As was the case for my family, some of these lessons, might have to be learned the hard way. I had no idea you were supposed to be well hydrated before blood work, until I stumbled upon the info online after a nurse was having a hard time finding my dad's vein. Again, one more very important and informative fact I would discover during one of my late night research sessions. I would have thought that exercise was a terrible idea for someone who is fighting an illness until our naturopath told us how important it was. This is another reason why I hope to get this book into as many hands as possible. I don't want you to be alone during this journey. If just one of my experiences is able to provide guidance and ultimately give you a sense of hope, then my dad's fight was worth it.

CHAPTER 11

THINGS FINALLY STARTED TO GET BAD

Minus two stints in the hospital for diverticulitis (not cancer related), my dad didn't really have too many issues that kept him from living a normal life. He would get tired a lot, but would nap when needed. He seemed invincible for almost two years.

If your loved one is currently battling cancer, then you already know – or are about to find out – that they need to go in for updated scans every few months. These scans will show progress of the cancer and indicate whether or not further treatments are needed. Sometimes they also result in those ugly ugly words of, "There's nothing more we can do."

Time and time again, I would take my dad for those

scans. I remember him joking about the awful taste of the liquid they made him drink before one of the tests. A week after the scan, I would take him in to get the results. Across the span of two years, those nervous days always ended with, "Everything looks great and let's continue with what we are doing" from his oncologist. My mom would sit at home or work frantically waiting for our phone call with the news. You could hear her sense of relief when I conveyed the message of, "It's all good."

My dad was doing so well that we planned and booked a family cruise for February of 2015. The entire family, ranging from grandparents to aunts and uncles were set to sail the Caribbean sea. Something we all hadn't done together in a long time. That was until….

Now the rest of this might be hard to read, but will show real examples of the true life and responsibilities of a caregiver.

It was late 2014, and once again another round of scans. During this time, my dad was on what's called 'maintenance chemotherapy' which meant going for chemo once every few weeks to keep everything in check. We went in for the results of the scans and this time, it wasn't good news. We found out that the cancer had spread to his brain fluid. This wasn't a good thing because radiation isn't as effective on cancerous brain fluid. But it was the only option. The doctor asked if we even wanted to try it—code for, *this might not work so you might as well live the weeks you have left as normal as possible or give it a shot and live with the effects of the radiation.* Without hesitation, my dad piped up and said, "Let's do it." A true fighter. He was now scheduled to undergo another ten rounds of radiation on his brain. And alas, his licence was once again stripped from him.

He completed the radiation like a champ. We had to wait a few weeks for a follow up scan to see if it had worked or not, but sadly we got our answer before then. In late November of 2014, we went to watch my nephew play hockey. After the game, and while we waited in the lobby for everyone, my dad turned to us and said something. We couldn't hear him, so he had to repeat himself. It was pretty much gibberish. He couldn't form any sentences and was having trouble speaking. We hoped it was just that he was exhausted and we took him home. Upon pulling into our driveway, the same thing happened again. Gibberish out of his mouth. So we took him straight to the hospital in fear that he might be having a stroke. It turned out that he didn't have a stroke but that the swelling in his head, on account of the cancer in his brain fluid, was pushing on his brain so much it was causing his speech to be slurred and incoherent. At the time, he was weaning off the steroid pills he was taking during his radiation. These pills were to help keep the swelling down. Almost immediately after taking another pill, his speech came back, and he seemed normal once again. He told me how scared he was. He realized he hadn't been making sense but didn't know how to fix it. This was the first time he showed he was frightened and it hurt to see.

The doctors wanted to keep him overnight for observation and to make sure they got him back to normal. Now, my dad loved his house. He loved sitting in his own chair, and sleeping in his own bed. He was not a fan of staying at the hospital but understood the severity of the situation. I stayed with him an hour after visiting hours and then was politely kicked out by the staff. Around 2am, we received a call from the hospital saying that my dad was causing a scene. All he wanted to do was go home and threatened the nurse to call me to come pick him up. I drove to the hospital and didn't know I was about to witness one of the hardest sights of my life. As the elevator opened on his floor, someone who looked like my dad was sitting in a chair at the front desk. His hospital gown still on, and bag fully packed. I approached this man and he angrily said, "Come on Jay, let's go." I say someone that looked like my dad because everything that was happening was *completely* out of character for him. I tried to explain why he was in the hospital, that the doctors and nurses were looking out for his best interest. He tried pushing me out of the way. I did my best to softly restrain his advances for the elevator. "Get the fuck out of my way. I'm going home," he said. It was the first time I had ever heard my dad use that kind of language. I felt like this wasn't my dad. I didn't know this man. I knew something wasn't right. The nurses called security as my dad continued to yell down the halls and aggressively curse towards every medical staff he crossed paths with. I told him that I would stay the night with him and we could go home in the morning. Security arrived to the floor and he thought it was the police coming to arrest him. "Good. Take me to jail. Better than this place," he fiercely expressed. I tried so hard to calm him down and I knew what was going to happen next. A nurse pulled out a needle, and gave me the eyes that said, "Is it OK if I do this?". I'm not sure if I regret my decision, but I haphazardly gave them the nod to go ahead and sedate my father. It quickly calmed him down and we walked him back to his room.

I found out that the nurses had given him a sleeping pill. Nothing out of the ordinary though because he was taking them at home, but this time it had a reaction with the steroid and made his mind fly off the handle. I went home with tears in my eyes that night. I was basically fighting someone who looked like my dad. It was a tough experience for me.

The next morning I picked him up and I had to explain everything that happened. He was extremely embarrassed and very apologetic. I told him not to worry about it, that I was just so happy to have him back home and that I was able to have a real conversation with my dad again. A couple days later, he bought a box of chocolates and had me bring them up to those nurses to say sorry. Even in times of despair, he still thought of others and wanted to make things right.

The hair that grew back on my dad's head would slowly start falling out, and the hairless staple that *is* cancer, had once again returned. His legs would start to get weaker which was a side effect of his medication. The steroid greatly diminished the muscle mass in his legs, causing him to slowly start needing a hand when getting up from a chair and assistance with walking. We eventually ended up getting him a walker and we had to put extra railings on the walls so he could get up and down the stairs. One day while he was showering, a situation I'd been anticipating (and dreading) happened. I could hear the water running as if he had turned off the shower head, and the water was now coming out of the shower faucet only. A standard practice of how my dad turns the shower off when finished. But the water didn't stop. It was running for about 20 seconds, which I knew was uncommon. I raced upstairs, and opened the door to find my dad laying in the tub. His legs had given out, and he had fallen backwards, hitting his back on the faucet causing it to switch from the shower head. Hot water spraying on his body, he couldn't get up. He was in pain and I think he was embarrassed. He was laying there naked, now knowing his life would require direct assistance everyday. I took him to the hospital to address his discomfort from the fall. Luckily, the only physical damage was a broken rib. Later that night, we had safety handles installed in our shower. One to hold while in there, and one to help him step in and out. The situation could have been so much worse.

We had a physiotherapist come to the house to work with my dad to try and build back the muscle in his legs. Even though we installed a bedside rail, circumstances had progressed to the point where he needed our assistance to get out of bed. If he needed to use the restroom, he needed our hand to get there. I was home with him during the day, so it wasn't a problem. He could just call my name if he needed something. But nights seemed to be a bit more challenging. He would need my help, but I would be fast asleep. So here's what I did: I went to Home Depot, and found a unique extension cord. On one end was the part you plug into the wall outlet, on the other end was a couple spots where you could plug things into it, and in the middle there was a small hand switch. The switch could cut the power or turn on whatever you had plugged into it. I made it so the switch was right beside my dad's pillow. We had the power to the lamp next to his bed turned on and plugged it into the extension cord. This way he could turn his lamp on or off with the switch next to his pillow. He no longer had to get out of bed, or reach over to turn it on. To help with the issue of getting our attention, I attached an additional extension cord to it, ran it directly to my room, and connected a lamp and radio to it. Any time he turned on the power, not only would his own bedside lamp turn on, but my lamp and a radio as well. Whether 2am or 4am, whenever he needed me I'd wake up. All he had to do was flick that switch and he knew I would be there to help him.

My dad's legs got so bad that he couldn't safely shower himself anymore. We got him a bath chair to sit on, and every morning, I would be in there helping him clean up. I never thought I would one day be bathing my dad. If it was five years earlier, even the thought of it would have probably made me queasy. But this was the man who made sure I was spotless as a baby. My father, who had bathed me numerous times as a toddler, now needed my help and I wasn't going to back down from that task. It's interesting how the cycle of life works. It was also the first time I had ever shaved someone else. My dad hated any sort of facial hair, which is surprising because he used to rock the best moustache. I didn't know how to shave someone else's face. What if I cut him? I was nervous but I put that aside to make him feel happy.

I can remember a time helping him into my van after taking him to purchase his weekly lotto tickets. As he was trying to get into the passenger seat, his legs gave way and I thankfully caught him before he fell onto the ground. I was holding my dad in my arms. At this point, he had lost a lot of weight and probably weighed somewhere around 140 lbs. As it turns out, lifting 140 lbs vs. lifting 140 lbs of motionless weight are two different things. I really struggled. I was bouncing him around. I believe his head may have hit the top of the door. I used whatever strength I had, to basically throw his body onto the seat, and then lift his legs into the car. I buckled him in, and then took a minute while I gasped for air.

The time had come to get the results of my dad's CT scan to see if the radiation on his brain was working. My normal procedure was to drive up to the hospital, let my dad off at the front door, and he would walk in and sit down while I went to park my van before meeting him in the lobby. This day was different. This time I drove up to the front door, got out of my van to grab a wheelchair, sit my dad in the chair, wheel him inside, and then I would go park my vehicle. It was liked I blinked and he went from walking on his own to sitting in a wheelchair.

I wheeled him into the doctor's office where we talked to his oncologist. She didn't waste any time to tell us that the radiation didn't work and his cancer was spreading more. "So I should keep doing the chemotherapy, right?," my dad hopefully asked. But I knew well enough that there wasn't much point. She told us it was up to him; that we could continue the maintenance chemo treatments but it wasn't going to help the brain. I can still remember the end of that appointment. Our oncologist got up, walked over to my dad, bent over and gave him a kiss on the cheek and said, "All the best." I took it as his kiss of death. Everything had been done to extend his life and soon it would be over.

It wasn't really the words I wanted to share with my mother that day. After two years of a somewhat normal life, it now seemed to be filled with daily moments of bad news.

Next would come a fall backwards while at the casino. My dad had hit his head on the ground so hard, paramedics had to stretcher him off to the hospital. He would then develop some sort of neurological pain in the side of his face. This pain, he said, felt like sharp knives cutting from his ear to his jaw, over and over. The doctors had put him on a medication for this, but it didn't seem to work. The pain would come at random times, and last about a minute or so. What seemed to help was when he held one of our hands during these episodes. They were so bad that he couldn't scream our names for help, so we had to improvise. We used baby monitors, and placed them beside his bed, and beside his favorite lazy boy chair. We could hear when he was in pain and rushed to his side to hold his hand through it. I'm not sure why clenching onto us helped him, but I didn't care. I was there to offer support any way I could.

It was struggle after struggle until the afternoon of January 30, 2015. I had to step out for a quick meeting but he assured me he was safe sitting in his chair and basically forced me to go. I then got a call from my mom saying she came home for lunch and didn't have the strength to get my dad up from the chair and was wondering when I would be home. This call quickly escalated to her calling an ambulance because my dad's legs had gotten so bad. My mom told me that while they were waiting for help, he leaned over to her and said, "I think I'm dying." I think right then and there, he had accepted what was to come next. It would be his last time in our home. And even though it's been two and a half years since that day, I just got choked up writing it.

I met them at the hospital and spent as many hours

as I could there over the next few weeks. I even remember bringing my dad his favorite chips and watching the Super Bowl with him.

I want to share a post I made and a photo I took on Super Bowl Sunday, February 1, 2015:

Came to the hospital to watch the Super Bowl with my Dad.

After a few tough days of intense fighting, it's great to see him up and excited to watch the game.

I have everything I need right now. My Dad, the game, and Doritos.

Magic happens when you never give up.

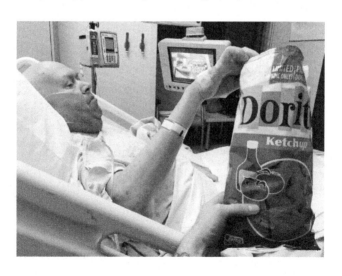

THINGS FINALLY STARTED TO GET BAD

My dad was now in the care of trained professionals. Some might say my job was done, but I knew being a caregiver was more than just doing specific things. It was about being there. It was about being beside him, so he wasn't alone. Nobody should be alone while fighting for their life and I still live with regret thinking about those nights my dad spent by himself in the hospital. I should have never listened to the visiting hours. I should have been there right beside him. There was a chair and my dad. That's all I needed. Getting over this is something I have to continue to work on.

After a few weeks of hospital care, the administrative staff and doctors explained to us that there wasn't much more they could do for my dad. Our best bet was to look at moving him to a hospice, which was another step I knew would come. He was all set to move on a Thursday afternoon, from hospital to hospice. We had arranged a patient transfer vehicle, and while my mom and I were heading up to the hospital to accompany him, we received a call to say that my dad had had a seizure. This was something new and the doctors wanted to keep him another day to monitor what was happening. When we got to the hospital, the doctors explained what happened – and it hit me. He had been having seizures for the past month and we had no idea. They told us that when they tried to communicate with him, he couldn't talk, and just stared with a silent daze to one spot in the room. It would take a few minutes before he would come to. I had witnessed this numerous times recently and thought he was just really tired and didn't want to talk. TV had taught me that seizures meant extreme and violent convulsions, combined with foaming at the mouth. I share this with you to be on the lookout for any abnormal behavior. This behavior wasn't that my dad was just exhausted, it was irregular electrical activity happening in his brain that was causing these episodes. I look back and think that it was situations like this that probably caused his legs to give out. I feel so bad that I didn't know, and passing on this information is something I strongly believe needs to be shared.

The staff at the hospice took such amazing care of my dad. They made it feel like a home and not a hospital. But it was a very sad feeling in there. This is where people came to die. My dad thought it was a rehab apartment and that once he got better, he would be going home. I didn't have the heart to tell him the truth. Maybe I was still holding onto hope that we could take him out of there and back into his own bed. But it came to a point where we physically couldn't care for him anymore. He needed the assistance of professionally trained staff and equipment our house wasn't fitted with. I can remember times my dad would be laying in his bed, the back angled up so he could comfortably watch television and a small bead of water would fall from the corner of his eye down to his cheek. I assumed it was his eyes getting watery from yawning, but the more I thought about it, it was probably a single tear of sadness. I think he knew what was happening and it made me feel so helpless.

So why tell you everything that I went through? As I said earlier in this book, I wasn't going to sugar coat anything. I wanted to show you exactly what I experienced. Now, this doesn't mean that these exact experiences are coming your way, but my hope is that you take these words and know that at some point, hard times are most likely ahead. The easy thing to do is put the responsibility on someone else, and the cowardly thing to do is run. I can't promise you enough, that you will feel a remarkable amount of regret if you decide to choose that path. I also promise you that when the time comes to reflect and look back, you'll be incredibly happy that you chose the path that led to being a witness of struggle and participating in ongoing heartache. I miss my dad so much, but what he taught me about life during his battle was more educational than any school or workshop could ever have been. Growing up, we were always very close, but I grew closer to him in those two years of illness, than I had my whole life. He became my best friend and I did the things I needed to do to make the man who meant the most to me happy. He fought for me, so I sure as hell was going to fight for him.

CHAPTER 12

MONEY VS. MEMORIES

It feels like I've been living in healthcare facilities over the last few months. I come home in the evenings just to sleep, and alas, my 6am alarm goes off, and I'm off again. Eating poorly, always exhausted, and spending what money I have left, on gas, coffees and whatever I need to make the people that mean the most to me, more comfortable.

Two years ago, I made the easy decision to basically become a full time caregiver for my family. This morning was spent with my dad, and this afternoon was spent at a different location with my grandfather. I'm broke.... I'm tired.... I have no life..... and I wouldn't have it any other way.

I haven't worked much in the last year or so. Haven't been able to take jobs I know would require a few days, nor have I been able to seek out new work. The opportunities are out there, but I prefer to spend time with my family.

I write this post, not looking for any sort of pat on the back, but to hopefully motivate those who might be questioning what to do about their situation, as well as provide reassurance to those who are doing the same as I, that they are doing the right thing.

I sat at my dad's bedside for about six hours this morning. He was probably sleeping for about five of them. Every so often, waking up to ask me to get him a drink of water, or to fix his sheets. I sat there wondering about the incredible or high paying jobs I was missing out on, but I also knew that there will always be time to make money, always be opportunities out there, but the days where I can get my dad a drink, or fix his sheets will soon come to an end. There's no amount of money that will replace these moments I have with him. Even though he's sleeping, I know he realizes I'm by his side, and he's not alone.

This brings me to now, where I spend my afternoons with my grandfather. Today he turns 89! Every year I bring him a balloon, birthday card, scratch tickets and a 6-pack of Labatt 50, although this year I had to bring him a 6-pack of his favorite donuts instead. Coming straight from seeing my dad, I am tired, hungry, and wound up what change I could find in my pocket to buy a chocolate bar for lunch. I read on Facebook about all the amazing and expensive things people are buying. The new, over-sized houses they are buying and the cars that the banks will take from them in four years. I look down at my chocolate lunch and realize how lucky I actually am. I might not have a ton of 'assets', but I got to celebrate my grandfather's 89th birthday with him today. The smile on his face as I walked in holding his balloon and gift, is what makes my decision to give up my life for them, worth it.

When I look back on all of this, I will never have one day of regret. I urge all of you to take a look at this "busy" life we all strive for and to take a look at what your end goal is. If it's money related, I promise you that you'll one day end up miserable.

Making money is way easier than making memories. You can always make money, but you might not always be able to make memories. I challenge you to cut back on your work this weekend, and spend it with your family and friends. Make someone dinner. Play video games with your kids. Go see your parents. Money doesn't care about us, so why do we care about it more than our families?

If family isn't on the top of your list, then happiness is definitely on the bottom.

This was a Facebook post that I wrote in March of 2015. At this time, my dad was in the hospice. About two years into my dad's journey, my grandfather started to become ill as well and was bedridden in a hospital. I was now caregiver for my two best friends, but I knew I was doing the right thing.

Here is another post I wrote on March 24, 2015 that deals with a very similar subject:

I've walked through the ravaged streets of Haiti, climbing over fallen trees, dodging burning cars all while Haitian rebels point their guns in my direction, yelling at me in a language I don't understand, which translated to 'Put your camera away or we'll shoot you.' I've driven cross-country with four other people, living in a cramped van, eating and drinking off of $4.00 a day, yet the hardest thing I've ever had to do is watch the two mentors in my life, the two men who taught me how to be a man, slip away to the next chapter of their lives, right in front of me.

I write this at the bedside of my dad, just as I finished helping him with his breakfast. It will probably be the only hour I see him awake today. He asked me what I did the previous night. Who won the curling event. And before he takes a bite, he needs to know that I already ate breakfast and offers a bite of his donut in case I still might be hungry. We then watch "The Price is Right" and make jokes about how awkward Drew Carey is, until his eyes become heavy and he falls back to sleep.

The room is warm, painted a grey shade, spotless, and smells like some sort of lavender the staff use to sanitize everything. My dad is comfortable, and I look back on the hour I spent with him today and smile. The "I feel embarrassed for him" comment about Drew Carey and the laugh we had will forever be etched into my mind; and that's something nobody can take away.

My morning and afternoon with my Dad would come to an end, and next up is to go spend some time with my grandfather. His advancing dementia and worsening condition have now moved him into a different ward. A ward where he's not allowed a TV in his room, has to use a punch code to get out the door and everything is restricted. I wasn't sure what to expect but upon entering his new room, the white walls, cold floor and emptiness reminded me of a jail cell. He was sitting up on the side of his bed, basically staring at the wall. My presence gave him a smile and a renewed sense of purpose. He was excited to see me but my mind wandered to a thought of "what would he be doing if I didn't show up? Is this how some people spend the last days of their lives, alone and sitting on the end of their bed?"

We sat and talked, and he recalled the fun days he had while living in Hamilton those many years ago. He was curious about how he got back home to

MY DAD GOT SICK

Saskatchewan. I had to explain to him that he was still living in Hamilton and that I was old enough to drive when he asked how I got there. I remember the days when I thought my grandfather was the smartest person I had ever met. The facts he knew and the knowledge that lived inside of him is what made him such a mentor and best friend in my life. He taught me how to be a listener and to be like glue; always collecting the most information you can get.

When I was younger, I had this dream I would one day buy my dad a 1950 Mustang, I would send my grandfather back home to his farm in Esterhazy, Saskatchewan and build him the biggest house ever............ but now I want to give them something more valuable and something I know they'll appreciate even more....... my time.

I think back on my morning spent bedside laughing with my dad. And I know he'll one day leave with that memory firmly planted inside of him. That I gave up whatever it was I had to do, to make sure he was OK.

And I think of the moment I just experienced with my grandfather.

His biggest struggle right now is that he can't focus and has lost the knowledge to finish the crossword puzzle that comes in our local paper. It was one of his favorite morning activities. I noticed he had started it. Got a few words but then gave up. I asked if he would like my help and that we could do it together. His eyes lit up and he was like a new man. I sat there for over an hour. Going over each clue with him, working as a team and soon half the puzzle was complete. I was twenty minutes away from missing the scheduled run I told myself I was to go on, but now, finishing this crossword with my grandfather was more important. The feeling of determination and focus we had, blocked out the screaming patient down the hall. I was now that screaming patient. Yelling out answers to the puzzle so that my grandfather would hear me. And we did it! The look on his face (as seen in the picture) when we completed that puzzle is something I'll have with me forever. I'll always cherish that proud look on his face.

This was last week.

The completed puzzle hasn't left his bedside and there isn't a soul in that hospital he hasn't told the story of doing the puzzle with his grandson. The big house in Saskatchewan wouldn't last forever, but when his time comes, he'll have this memory to bring onward with him and so will I.

I write this in hopes to help answer the question that some of us may have: "What can I do for them?" When looking to comfort or take care of our loved ones, our first reaction is "What can I buy them?" Material possessions only offer a brief moment of satisfaction and we all get over it. I hope this will make you realize how valuable time is. It's the one thing we can never get back. You lose money, you can make more. Your car breaks down, you can get another one. You spend time with those who mean the most to you, and that's the most valuable thing you can offer to anyone.

I strongly feel that my dad has exceeded the doctor's odds and that my grandfather is still around because my family has continually gave them the one medicine that can't be stopped.... Love.

My dad knows that we will come everyday to see him and he looks forward to that. My grandfather knows visitors are on the way and he can't wait. I don't care what any experts say, a family's love is the best medicine you can give someone in need.

Without love, you have nothing to look forward to. Spend time with those you love, and you'll love the time spent with them.

It's now May of 2017 as I sit here and write this. I didn't get back to work full-time until January of 2016 and it was a terrible business year for me. I brought in about $17,000 in sales, and coupled with my expenses, I claimed a nice big loss. I was almost starting off at square one, trying to get clients back while working to build and update a new portfolio. After all was said and done, I found myself in about $90,000 of debt, desperately trying to climb back to zero. If I didn't take that time off to take care of my dad, I know I would be making great money right now, living in my own house without debt, and I'd have probably toured the world multiple times. But on any day of the week, I can go to a travel agent and book a trip. What I can't do is go to a store and book time with my dad. I knew our time was limited and I did everything in my power to maximize that. But even with all my accumulated debt, I sit here today, knowing that I made the right decision. I know in my heart that one day, I'll be back on top in my business, and I'll have my best friend looking down on me everyday. Let me tell you that being this much in debt, really, really sucks. There's days where I question if I'll ever get out of it and at times it pushes my anxiety levels to new heights. But I don't what to live my life with regret. I don't want to know what it would be like, day after day, to question your decisions and how it could have negatively affected those closest to you. I fear those anxiety levels would be a million times worse. I can't imagine a world where someone would choose money over memories, but unfortunately it exists.

If there is one thing I hope you take away from this book, it's that every sacrifice you make to give time to your loved one will be the best decision you'll ever make. I may not be a rich man, but I am wealthy beyond words. Once you stop associating 'rich' with 'money' and start looking at how rich you are in family, friends, and the time you spend together, money will take on a whole new meaning. I don't regret one single thing about giving up two and a half years and I know how much I've learned and grown from it. I also know how much regret some people are currently feeling because they put the almighty dollar and visions of climbing that corporate ladder ahead of family. Don't be that person. Making money is so much easier than making memories with someone who is gone.

The look of joy and happiness on my grandfather's face after we completed that crossword puzzle.

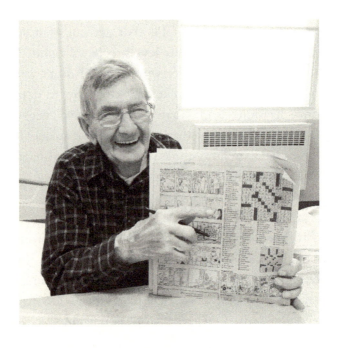

CHAPTER 13

HE'S GONE... BUT THE JOURNEY CONTINUES

It was the words I knew were coming one day, but that I didn't want to believe. It was a Thursday evening when I got a call asking me not to go too far because my dad's breathing was getting very bad. I quickly rushed to the hospice around 10pm, sat bedside with him, and held his hand as my brother and uncle also looked on. My mom waited until we arrived and then went home to get some sleep. She couldn't bear to see him like that. Her love was quickly slipping into his next life.

Every hour or so, my dad would open his eyes and stare at us. His condition had paralyzed his speech but his eyes narrated everything. He was saying his goodbyes.

This would happen over and over throughout the night. His eyes would open, look at all of us, and slowly close – a memory that will last with me forever. We were communicating only with vision and it was a magical moment. His look read as, "Hey, Jay, I love you. Thank you for all you have done. Go kick some ass in this world. I'll always be watching." Mine said, "Thank you, Dad. Thank you for everything." We connected as only father and son could.

At 8am my mom showed up. She realized she needed to be there and told me to head home to get some sleep, promising she would update me on what was happening. A few hours later, on April 3, 2015, I received that terrible call and with a brave breath, my mom uttered the words, "He's gone." I quickly dressed and headed back to the hospice to be with my family and to give my dad one last kiss and say goodbye. I asked my mom how he went and it all made sense. My mom – bedside – held his hand as he struggled to breathe, and just like with us, he opened his eyes. Their eyes locked and I can only imagine the emotion in that moment. Happiness and sadness on a level some of us might never know. He was saying goodbye to the girl of his dreams and she was saying goodbye to her high school sweetheart. My mom told him it was OK to go, and soon after, he was gone. I never fully understood why he kept opening and closing his eyes while I was there until I heard that story. He knew he was close to his last breath but held on until he could say goodbye to everyone that filled his heart with love. He was waiting for my mom.

This was my first time dealing with the death of a loved one right in front of me. My prior experiences with death came from what movies told me it would be like. Time and time again, films depict somebody fighting a terminal illness via an Oscar worthy scene; a scene where the patient offers his/her one last piece of advice before they pass. Ninety-nine percent of the time that advice has to do with family. Either the loved one will tell the ill person, "It's okay to go, I'll take care of everyone", or the ill person will urge their loved one to spend more time with his or her family before closing their eyes and fading away.

I wish I could tell you that I had this Hollywood moment with my dad. But I didn't. Maybe I'm bitter because I had hoped it would happen, but I'm learning that carving up expectations based on the movies you watch might lead you to disappointment if they don't occur. Movies do tell some truths about death and dying, but it's quite different when you're actually living through it. There was no Hollywood ending for me. There was no Oscar worthy scene. I never got it, but what I did get was 32 years of oscar worthy moments with my dad. I feel so lucky that I got that much time with him. You could maybe say that my

Hollywood ending was a silent film but one that will replay in my mind over and over.

Since I had been sharing his journey online, I felt like I needed one more post to give Dad the send off he deserved. I waited a day so we could be together as a family and then I made it public.

Written on April 4, 2015:

> *We often like to admire those UFC mixed martial artists, boxers, and even our crazy Canadian hockey players, as they step into their ring time after time and show their bravery as we deem them 'fighters'. We associate them with such terms as: 'confident', 'fearless', 'muscular', 'heroic', and 'courageous'. We put them high on our list of icons we look up to for having such traits.*
>
> *Now let's look at my dad for a second. For those that know him, you might associate, 'small', 'quiet', 'shy', 'delicate', and 'opposite of muscular' as traits he possesses. But I have no problems putting my dad at the same level if not higher as those 'fighters' we all admire.*
>
> *On March 5th, 2013, my dad and my family were given the dreadful news that his cancer was so severe that it would take his life in nine months to a year.*

In that nine months to a year, I got to witness my dad turn from a shy, timid person, to an individual I was confident could knock out Muhammad Ali. And on March 6th, 2014 he would start his victory lap the doctors said wouldn't exist. He gave the middle finger to cancer and I saw my dad reach a goal they said wasn't possible.

As of yesterday morning, around 11:00 am, and after 394 days of a victory lap, my dad decided to call it a day and left this world.

As hard as it is not to be sad, I am smiling from ear to ear at how proud I am of my Dad. In these last two plus years, he's taught me how to be a winner, how to be successful and how to prove the experts wrong.

I can go on and on, stating amazing quality after amazing quality that my dad had deep down inside, but the one thing he demonstrated time and time again, was love. There wasn't a more loving person on this earth. He would do anything for his family and I truly believe that it was love that kept him around so long. No medicine could compare. No treatment was equal. The knockout punch my dad had, was love.

I will miss my dad deeply, and promise to bring his full story to light one day. I want to tell the story of a David, who turned into a Goliath, but won.

MY DAD GOT SICK

Even though my dad was a quiet man, if you throw a few rum & Cokes in him, he'll have you laughing all night. Joke after joke. If you are out this evening, raise a rum & Coke in his honor. It was one thing he had to give up when he started his two year journey and I know he's up there right now, throwing a few back with his family who was waiting for his arrival. Dad, I look forward to the day where we can once again share a drink. So until then, please keep a cold one for me in the fridge and I'll see you soon. Love you!

It's the day I knew was slowly approaching, and if your loved one has a terminal diagnosis, I'm sure you might be expecting it too. There's no other way to say it, other than it sucks. It really does. It was also the first time in my life that I felt like I had lost. As a caregiver, winning to me meant that I would find a way to cure my dad and he would be with me for many, many more years. But I couldn't cure him and I felt defeated. To make matters even worse, a few weeks later, my grandfather passed away. Gone were the two father figures in my life; the two people who I went to for advice or just to relax and have a beer with. In a matter of weeks, they were both gone.

I easily went into a depression and my anxiety skyrocketed. I started to ignore some of the closest people around me. My relationship at the time was struggling and I definitely wasn't myself. It took many months but I pushed through. I had written a few pages of this book soon after his death but I stopped for a long time. I wasn't in the right frame of mind and I needed some help. I thought I was always sick. I found myself going to the doctor and hospital over and over, thinking every pain I had was cancer. I mean, why wouldn't it be, right? Seeing how many people were in the chemo clinic every time got me to believe that it's not *if* you'll be diagnosed with cancer, but *when*. It was really baffling to see how many people were sick. And even though my dad was gone, I was still fighting that disease — 'The Caregivers Disease'.

I had burnt myself out by focusing on taking care of too many people and forgetting to take care of myself. My stress levels were at an all time high and I knowingly wasn't much fun to be around. I had to take time to work on myself as you will have to do as well. They say 'Time heals all wounds', but the same people also say, 'The customer is always right'. Both are sayings we know to be complete B.S. Sure, time might heal a physical ailment, but the emotional scars that become buried deep into your mind after witnessing a loved one suffer will never completely heal. You just find ways to cope with it.

Just the other day, I had a psychologist friend question the possibility of a post traumatic stress disorder (PTSD) diagnosis while she witnessed me hesitantly answer my cell phone. There are a few things in my life I still need to fight through and work on. During my dad's journey, one of the scariest things that used to happen was when our house phone would ring. It was the phone number the doctor's had to get a hold of my dad or the family. Whenever that ringer went off, and the call display read 'private caller', we knew it wasn't good news. I dreaded hearing that sound and to this day, whenever I hear the phone ring, I instantly think it's bad news. *It's 2017, why would someone call me when they can just send a text?* is what my mind tells me. It must be bad news. And while saying hello, I prep myself for what is to come next. Ninety-nine percent of the time, it's nothing bad and I made my anxiety levels rise for no reason. The psychologist explained that this thought process is very similar to individuals who serve in the military and come home and hear thunder during a storm. They relate it to the gun fire, and it ignites their fight or flight response.

Do you remember that fresh, glowing red v-neck tee shirt that still had the price tag on it I talked about in the first paragraph of the March 5, 2013 chapter? The first thing I did when I got home was rip up that shirt and throw it in the garbage. It was the shirt's fault that we got bad news that day. It was the shirt's fault that my dad was going to die. I had convinced myself that it, alone, was the cause of this bad luck and to this day, I have never worn a red piece of clothing. I have never used a red pen, and I now go as far as to avoid items if they come in a label or packaging that is red in color. Some might say I do this subconsciously, but I would say I have willingly trained my psyche to perceive this color as the color of the devil and bad luck.

To continue this trend, I am forever haunted by the number 35. We got that terrible news on March 5, the third month, and the fifth day: 35. I see it everywhere. When I was in Las Vegas, I went to my dad's favorite casino to have a drink for him, and sure enough, I look at the address: 3535 S Las Vegas Blvd. Receipts totaling $35, licence plates on rental cars being R-35, and here's the craziest one: my grandfather passed away on May 8, 2015. I decided to count how many days that was after my dad passed, and sure enough, 35! Some have tried to convince me that it's a good sign but I'm still struggling with that thought. How could March 5th be a good thing. Coincidentally, I write these words at 35 years of age.

I watch the mood of my mom everyday. I can tell she is sad. I can feel she is lonely. She lost the person she was supposed to live and grow old with and now she is left to do that by herself. I tell most people that I'm happy, but deep down, I don't think I am. I still struggle with what I witnessed.

I tell you about this sadness and struggles because it's true and it's something you very well might experience. But it's OK. Opening up like this is hard for me but I want you to know that you aren't alone. You might deal with the loss of a loved one better than me, or maybe worse, but do know that the grieving process takes time and the only thing that will make it worse is rushing it. It took me almost two years to finally get back to writing this book. Two years that I needed to reflect and grieve. And there is nothing wrong with that. My PTSD, the color red, the number 35, are all things I continue to work on personally. I know one day they will all be a thing of the past but I'm not dashing for that finish line. I will take my time to make sure I do it right. The one thing that seems to help is writing. Maybe deep down this is another reason why I'm writing this book. As much as its intention is to help you, maybe it's helping me just as much. Maybe these words are my medication. Point is, do whatever it is you have to do to get through this pain. Never be embarrassed to seek professional help, never be too weak to call a friend just to talk, and never feel like you are alone.

This is why this book has taken me so long to write. The journey doesn't stop with death, that's only the halfway point. The story continues and my personal fight lives on.

I write this on August 6, 2017, 856 days after my dad's passing.

I thought I would have been able to write this book within a week of that day. I mean, the stories have already happened. They are in my head and all I had to do was get pen to paper. But what I didn't realize, was what comes after.

The pain is still here. The emptiness still exists, and I sometimes struggle knowing I can no longer turn to my dad for advice. Just last night, a song came on that reminded me of him and I shed a few tears. My tears won't go away and I don't think they should. I believe the more you cry, the more you loved.

The hardest times that lay ahead are those special days that your loved one will miss for the first time. For me, it was my birthday – a day I'd been dreading since his passing. Here is a Facebook post I made on May 28, 2015:

On a day that brings such happiness, I can't help but feel like there's something missing.

This is the first time I didn't wake up to a birthday French toast breakfast made by my Dad. If it was a work day, he would prepare it before he left, and make sure it stayed nice and warm for when I woke up. If I wasn't there, he would somehow get it to me. It's a different feeling this morning, but I also feel great joy for the time I had with him and the friends and family I currently have around me.

I have numerous photos, numerous memories, but the one thing I've been missing, was hearing my Dad's voice.

Last night I went through some old video footage, and crazy enough the first tape I found, had a clip of my birthday party from 1992, and my Dad was in it. I am so grateful that this exists and that my parents were memory hoarders, just like me. I know him and my Grandpa are up there having a party for me today.

His voice was the one thing that I missed the most about him. It felt so nice to hear it once again. As a photographer, I understand how powerful a photo can be, but you will never understand the power of someone's voice until it's no longer there.

I had avoided Father's Day 2015 as best I could. It went from such a special day, to just a Sunday for the first time in my life. I felt alone and did my best to keep myself busy that day and shut myself from social medial to bypass all the fun everyone was having with their dads. But looking back, I missed an opportunity. I missed a chance to honor the man who I routinely celebrated every fathers day before that. I promise you that avoiding things going forward will only bring you more pain.

Father's Day of 2016, I had the unbelievable opportunity to be traveling through Norway. And on that sacred Sunday, I had a moment with my dad that nobody can take from me.

Here is the post I made on June 19, 2016:

There's nothing more I wanted to do in life than make my Dad proud.

He was a quiet man. Never did show much emotion but I always knew he was my biggest supporter.

I'm not much of a religious person, and my thoughts on whether heaven is real or not are mixed, but if it is, this was the closest I've been to him in a long time and it was something I needed to feel. I was above the clouds and got to have my own time alone with him. I updated him on everything new in my life but he already knew that.

Call me crazy, but I had one of the biggest ideas of my life come to me at that moment. Norway has motivated me beyond words. Dad, I know you're proud of me, but even grander things are on the rise. I promise you. I miss you but I know you're always a hike up to the clouds away.

I want to send a Father's Day greeting to all those amazing Dads out there. Dads rule!

I had no idea that that moment, the photo that was taken during it, and that experience would one day grace the cover of the book I was writing. This book.

Some people might say that I was wasting my time and that I was just talking to the clouds but I did something that genuinely made me feel better. I urge you to do what makes you feel good, and to do what works for you. If you believe that you're just talking to thin air, then don't do it. But if you truly believe your loved one is listening from above, I promise you it's helpful.

I've had a few people tell me that this book needs a 'Moving On' chapter, and quite frankly, this is why this paragraph exists. But to be honest, I don't think I will ever move on. To me, moving on means to forget about the past. It means forgetting about the individual who helped me become the incredible person I am today. I will never forget about my dad and instead of moving on, I want to call it moving forward with the strength and wisdom that came from dealing with tragedy. I want to take everything I witnessed and turn that into a positive. Moving on is something that I'm still figuring out; it may require more than just one chapter one day.

> *"I learned that courage was not the absence of fear, but the triumph over it. The brave man is not he who does not feel afraid, but he who conquers that fear."* - Nelson Mandela

I had nothing to prepare me for the death of my father and I had no personal stories of life after death to lean on. I'm doing this alone, but I want *my* footsteps to lead you down the path of conquering what lies ahead.

CHAPTER 14

PLEASE, DON'T FORGET TO TAKE CARE OF YOURSELF

My logic during my dad's illness was that the more time I spent taking care of him, the better he would be. I sacrificed my own sleep, my appetite, my social life, and so much more. I ended up losing ten pounds out of nowhere. It wasn't until one day where I physically couldn't get out of bed that I realized every ounce of energy in my body was being used on others and that it made me a prisoner to physical activity. It was that day that I looked in the mirror and realized I, too, needed to make some changes. How could I tell my dad to eat healthy, when I wasn't? A diet of Subway and Doritos wasn't the wisest of ideas, and I knew that. I started to consume more fruits and vegetables. I made sure to get the sleep I needed, to keep my body well rested. I started morning meditations that have significantly helped with my anxiety issues. I exercise daily to help ignite the biochemical process known for releasing our 'happy hormones'. I did my best to not only cut out the negative people in my life, but to surround myself with positive and supportive individuals. I feel it's so important to continually surround yourself with people. Being alone is not a good idea and I found out the hard way. But none of this was easy. To take time for myself, required taking time away from my dad. I talk about how I was the primary caregiver for my dad, and although true, I can't forget to mention how important of a role my mom and brother played in this. It was only because of them, that I was able to spend some time taking care of myself. If you have the option to do this as a team, I would highly recommend doing so. The healthier you stay, and the more energy you have, the better decisions you will make and the better care you will be able to provide for your loved one. I never let my dad know that I was burning out. It would have made him feel even worse. So I made it my mission to get better. For him, AND for me.

When you're on an airplane during the pre-takeoff safety briefing, you're told that if the cabin pressure is lost while in flight, oxygen masks will drop and you are to put yours on before you help your child with theirs. That's nice to 'recommend', but you and I both know that we are making sure our children are safe before we even think about putting on that mask. This was my exact thinking with my dad, only I forgot to put on my mask altogether. Take care of your loved one, but remember you deserve a mask too.

CHAPTER 15

WHAT TO DO NOW

I applaud you for making your way to the end of this book. I can only imagine how some of my stories may have sparked emotions that you may or may not have been ready to deal with. Life as a caregiver comes with such ups and downs. If you look at it as a job, it will be a time of sadness and disappointment. But if you're able to see above that and pull some positives from this, you'll absolutely bear witness to some incredibly magical moments.

Surprisingly, things became a lot easier when I finally accepted that my dad would one day not be here anymore. That day where you will have to call upon all your strength, and accept the fact that your loved one will no longer be with you, might come soon for you as well. But until then, you have a choice to make. You have the choice as to how you spend your time. You have the choice to reach out for personal assistance if you think you need it. And you have the choice to take these words and use it as motivation to explore alternative medicines and different methods to keeping your loved one healthy and around longer. Will it work? I can't say for sure, but I do know with 100 percent certainty, that doing nothing *won't*. The decision from here on out is ultimately in your hands. I can only tell you what I did and I hope my goal of inspiring you to want to do the same, works.

Being a caregiver was the hardest thing I've ever had to do. I don't really like to call it a 'job', because to me, the definition of a job is something someone does, that they don't like, for which they get paid to do. There are some really tough times ahead. You will get tired. You will get frustrated. And you will feel lonely. There were actually a few times that my dad and I got into an argument during his journey: me questioning if he had given up, which turned into a yelling match that I later felt incredible guilty for. But things like this might happen, and I feel as though it's quite normal. All I had to do was apologize and thank him for what he was doing and things were back to normal.

It's currently August of 2017 as I finish writing this book. I'm sitting outside, on my laptop, enjoying a cool summer day. But, just like I said in the start of this book, who cares. I told myself I would conclude these words once I thought there was adequate information to bring you forward on your journey. I put myself in those shoes I wore in early 2013, and asked myself what I would have wanted to know.

There will come a time when someone close to you, will unfortunately need these words as well. It's an inevitable part of the world we live in. I ask that when you pass along this book to them, you also pass on your own experiences, advice, and friendship. You know how much you needed a friend to check in on you every now and then, so be that friend for others when the time comes.

This was intended to be short. I wanted it to be finished in one sitting and I hope you were able to accomplish that. If you don't agree with some of the methods I used in the book, that's perfectly fine. Try and come up with your own. Research, research, and research. But most importantly, spend time. Time is the overarching theme in my words for a reason. We aren't all doctors, we aren't all healers, but the one thing we all have in common, is that we have the powerful ability to love. Promise me that you will not only spend the time, but love the time you spend with the person who needs it most right now. Because, depending on your definition, you can be witness to unimaginable daily miracles.

I wish you all the best on this journey.

He was my dad. He was a brother, son, husband, friend, high school sweetheart, cousin, and grandfather. His name was and will always be Darryl Perry. I love and miss you dad. I know you never doubted me, but I told you I would get your story out one day and that it would be used to help others. You still inspire me. Thank you for everything. I'll see you one day. Have a cold beer ready for me. Love Jay.

ABOUT THE AUTHOR

As a full-time photographer from Canada, Jay Perry has travelled the country and beyond to capture the moments and memories that matter. Following a photo trip to Haiti in 2010 – mere months after the devastation of the earthquake that shook its capital city – Jay discovered his passion for helping others and has since dedicated his time and talent to numerous charitable efforts while founding his own establishment aptly named Friends With Hearts which acts and operates as a global community of friends working together to restore the magic of Christmas for families in need.

For a closer glimpse into Jay's life, check out www.jayperry.ca, www.friendswithhearts.com, or his personal Instagram @jayperry

A piano has 88 keys.

Made in the USA
Monee, IL
20 March 2022